FLATTEN THAT BELLY, TRIM THOSE THIGHS:
The Leptin Sensitivity Enhancement Eating Plan

Editing by Maria D. Laso
Graphic design and layout by Kay Kaminski

Printed and bound in the United States of America.

Visit www.eduardodias.com.

Table of Contents

Introduction

Thank you for purchasing the **Flatten That Belly, Trim Those Thighs** eating plan.

This plan is the result of more than fifteen years of hands-on experience helping people achieve optimum weight and health through nutrition and exercise. It is a combination of the most effective diets I have come across in all my years of personal training and nutrition advising.

Eating properly is one of the most important things you can do for yourself. Beyond helping you achieve your desired weight and good health, eating correctly will have a positive effect on your mood and energy throughout the day, in your quality of sleep, and even in your ability to think clearly.

One of the most important realizations I have had by studying different diets is that no single diet works for everybody. We are as unique inside as we are outside: No two people's nutritional requirements are exactly alike. That's why the most effective approach I have found blends the best of the best while allowing room for your individual requirements.

I also realized that for a person to stick long-term with an eating plan, the plan has to be adaptable to the person's lifestyle, not the other way around.

Yes, this goes against what you may have heard from other nutrition experts. Conventional wisdom is that you must change to a healthy lifestyle to succeed at a diet. Although I agree that each of us should lead a healthy lifestyle, I add this caveat: If a diet doesn't work for a person who really tries, it's the diet, not the person, that failed. Extremely restrictive diets are bound to fail for most people because there is a limit to how much a person can change, maintain that change, and still be happy.

Some people prefer to eat out; some love to cook at home. If I told the first type of person that cooking is the only way to success, she would eventually give up and probably be miserable until she did. If I told the cook that he should stay out of the kitchen, he too would be doomed to failure and unhappiness.

I realized I need an eating plan that allows restaurant-eaters to eat healthfully while also being adaptable to those who would prefer to prepare their own meals. Likewise, someone on a budget needs an affordable plan.

A truly effective eating plan has to be flexible to fit every need, taste and lifestyle. Even those who have all of their meals delivered can achieve results with this plan, and you don't have to be a chef or a king to succeed.

Leptin Sensitivity Enhancement

One of the most important factors to health—including achieving and maintaining a healthy weight—is your body's ability to burn fat.

In The Rosedale Diet, Dr. Ron Rosedale puts it perfectly: *Eating fat doesn't necessarily make you fat and unhealthy…not being able to burn fat does.*

Of course the amount and type of fat you eat will greatly influence your ability to burn fat. That's one focus of the **Flatten That Belly, Trim Those Thighs** eating plan. The bottom line is, to achieve your ideal weight and ideal health, your body must be good at burning fat.

The bad news is, yes, your body can lose its ability to burn fat efficiently. The good news is that ability can be regained.

So how do we become "good" at burning fat?

Leptin is the answer.

Leptin is a hormone, a chemical messenger that establishes communication between body and brain. It is produced by white fat cells (the fat that accumulates on the **abdomen, buttocks and thighs**). Leptin has two main functions that make it the single key element in your ability to burn fat and maintain a healthy weight.

1. When you eat, leptin signals to your brain that you have had enough and that you are no longer hungry. Basically, it tells you to stop eating.
2. Leptin tells your brain when your body has stored enough fat and should begin burning fat for energy.

However, the key to burning fat and to controlling appetite is *not* to produce more leptin.

No, the answer is to get very good at *responding* to leptin. When your body consistently produces too much leptin, your brain becomes resistant to its messages.

An overweight person who has excessive white fat cells producing too much leptin has plenty in the bloodstream, but the brain can't perceive it. The message is that the body is starving. The brain is saying, "Eat more and conserve the little fat you have left!"

The solution is not to produce more leptin. The answer is to develop--or redevelop--your ability to respond to leptin. That's what Leptin Sensitivity Enhancement (LSE) is about.

The Seven Rules of LSE

How do you eat to enhance your sensitivity to leptin?

By observing the seven rules of Leptin Sensitivity Enhancement.

These easy-to-follow rules will guarantee your nutritional success by ensuring that you eat to maximize sensitivity to leptin. When you follow the LSE rules, your body becomes a self-regulating, fat-burning machine, very healthy and very good at maintaining a healthy weight, just as it is naturally supposed to be.

LSE allows you to customize your eating to individual tastes and lifestyle preferences, making it easier to stick with healthy eating habits as you discover your unique nutritional requirements. It's okay to eat out while following the LSE rules. If you love to cook, you can use the rules as guidelines in the kitchen.

No matter your preference, what foods you like, what lifestyle you lead, you can easily incorporate the LSE rules into your life.

Before you know it, healthy eating becomes natural and effortless.

1. Eat protein, carbohydrates, and fat in every meal.

This is a cornerstone of healthy eating, one of the most basic yet important things you can do. Simply put, the human body is made mostly of protein, fat and water and is fueled by burning carbohydrates and fat. Those four nutrients--water, protein, carbohydrates, and fats--are called **macronutrients** because they make up the bulk of our diet (micronutrients are vitamins and minerals, which we need in small amounts). Assuming you are drinking plenty of water, every meal should provide you with those other three essential nutrients—carbs, protein, fats. These three macronutrients work together for optimal utilization.

Fat slows your body's absorption of sugar. By eating fat with carbohydrates, you help keep blood sugar from getting too high too fast, which would make your body produce excessive insulin and, in turn, promote fat storage. The body synthesizes protein better when it is consumed with carbohydrates.

If you skip one of those macronutrients in a meal, you are not only depriving yourself of essential nutrients but also hindering the process of using those nutrients.

That doesn't mean that you have to eat high amounts of those three at every meal. As you will see in Rule No. 7, each person needs different amounts of each macronutrient; that can also vary between meals.

2. Wait five to six hours between meals. Eat three meals a day.

This is another cornerstone of successful healthy eating--and where I diverge from the consensus among most dietitians and nutritionists today.

At the time of this writing, the most common advice is to "eat five to six small meals a day, three to four hours apart." I disagree.

Although it may sound good theoretically, I believe this recommended pattern too often leads to overeating and a body unable to burn fat properly.

Unless you have a metabolic condition, such as diabetes or a poorly functioning liver, I believe you should eat three regular-size meals a day, five to six hours apart.

This is one of the most important steps to achieve ideal weight and optimal health and to condition your body to burn fat for energy. It also should make it easier to stick with your eating plan.

When you eat a well-balanced meal with carbohydrates, protein and fat, your body does three things with those calories, in this order:

• "Fills up" your bloodstream with glucose and fat to be used immediately as energy.
• Stores some calories (from protein and carbs) in your liver and muscles in the form of glycogen. Your liver can store 90-110 grams of glycogen (the equivalent of about three to four hours of normal activity). Your muscles can store 250-400 grams of glycogen.
• Stores the rest of the calories as fat in fat cells around your body.

For three to four hours after a meal, your body will convert the glycogen you stored in your liver into glucose and release it into your bloodstream to be used as energy. (The glycogen stored in your muscles can't be converted into glucose, but it will be used by the muscles themselves.)

When the glycogen in your liver is almost depleted, which takes three to four hours after eating, your body delves into its fat reserves, moving that fat into your bloodstream to be used for energy.

If you eat before that time, your body again will fill your liver with glycogen and use that for energy, never going into fat storage. That's why it's important to wait five to six hours between meals. It's after the third hour that your body goes into high-fat-burning mode.

Small meals change the timing on that process by not completely filling your glycogen reserves; your body is forced to tap into storage sooner. If a regular meal fills up your glycogen storage for three to four hours, then it follows that a small meal will give you about two hours. If you eat six small meals every three hours, you are at high-fat-burning mode for one hour each four times a day, as opposed two hours each twice a day.

The problem is that in reality, being able to have six healthy, well-balanced, small meals every day is completely unrealistic for most people. Because "under-eating" is not our natural instinct, many who eat several small meals are always a bit unsatisfied. That or they simply end up overeating what turns out to be six regular meals instead.

It is **a lot** of work to plan and prepare those six little meals every day, if they are going to be truly healthy, well-balanced meals. Suddenly it's three hours later and you have nothing healthy around, so you reach for whatever is available, and that's usually not good.

In theory, eating small meals every three hours would be just as good as eating a full meal every five to six hours, but *in reality* for most people this approach is a recipe for failure.

Right about now you might be wondering about when you get to snack.

No snacking between meals!

Snacking is one of the worst things you can do if you want to be healthy, because it will delay or even halt the fat-burning process. The minute you snack, your liver will fill with glycogen again, and you won't go into a fat-burning mode until that glycogen is gone. Depending on how soon you eat again, or how much you snacked, you might not go into fat burning mode at all.

For some people, the idea of not snacking between meals is almost unthinkable. The truth is, however, if you eat a regular, satisfying meal—complete with protein, carbohydrate, and fat—and provided you don't have a metabolic problem, you should have no problem waiting five to six hours before eating again. The problem for some is that they have gotten so used to eating all the time that their bodies have lost the ability to tap into fat stores for energy. That's why they have to continuously refill their glycogen storages by snacking. The good news is that with the LSE rules, you can change that.

Diabetics and people with health concerns who need to eat small meals three to four hours apart, should check with their doctor before starting this plan. Generally speaking, everything here will apply with the exception of the size of the meals and waiting five to six hours between meals.

Here is how you make it more doable: put together regular size meals, split them in ½ and eat each ½ three to four hours apart. This way you won't have to come up with five to six different meals every day, and you'll still have all your healthy, balanced meals. Again, check with your doctor. But that is how over the years my diabetic clients were able to adjust their eating.

3. Limit carbohydrates and saturated fat intake.

Carbohydrates

Generally in our society we tend to eat way too much carbs. Depending on metabolism and activity level, some may need more carbs than others. Still, as a rule, everybody should watch carb intake.

Carbs are more easily converted into body fat than are monounsaturated fats, polyunsaturated fats or proteins. In other words, you are much more likely to gain weight and have adverse health consequences from overeating carbs than from overeating protein and "good" fats.

It's a simple equation: Your body can store only so much carbs as glycogen--90 to 110 grams in your liver and 250 to 400 grams in your muscles. Once glycogen stores are full, anything more will be stored as fat.

You would have to eat a lot of low-starch vegetables to get too much carbs. If you stay away from fruit juices and sodas, stick to the carbs on the food table, and minimize or avoid starchy carbs, you should be fine.

To make it simple, I have listed which foods are carbs, and which of those are "good" or "bad" carbs.

1. **Low- or non-starch vegetables.** Good; eat as much as you want.
2. **Fruits.** Good in moderation.
3. **Whole grains and moderate starch vegetables.** Okay in small amounts for most. If you are trying to lose weight, avoid these at first; later you can add small amounts and see how your body reacts.
4. **Refined grains and high-starch vegetables.** Avoid.
5. **Candies, soda, fruit juices.** Strongly avoid.

Saturated Fat

First and foremost, let me be clear about one thing: *Eating fat is necessary.*

Fat is one of the macronutrients: Your body is made of water, protein, and fat. Every cell in your body has fat. The cell membrane of every cell in your body is largely made of fat. Fat is also necessary for the transportation of fat-soluble vitamins.

However, not all fats are the same. There are three types of fat that you should consume: monounsaturated, polyunsaturated, and saturated—although not in equal amounts.

Monounsaturated and polyunsaturated (especially omega-3) fats are easily used as energy, while saturated fat is easily converted to body fat and stored in the body, typically in the belly on men and on the hips for women.

Therefore, although you should consume some saturated fats, you should keep that consumption in check. Saturated fat should be about 20 percent of your total fat intake. In other words, 80 percent of your fat intake should be in the form of monounsaturated and polyunsaturated fats (especially omega-3).

In general, saturated fat is solid at room temperature and comes from animal sources. A simple way to keep your saturated-fat intake low is to cook only with vegetable oils, particularly olive oil, high-oleic (high-heat) sunflower oil, high-oleic (high-heat) safflower oil, or avocado oil.

Also, choose low-fat dairy and lean cuts of meat. If you stick to chicken and fish, limiting red meat and pork, you should be okay. Of course, there are some leaner cuts of red meat and lean pork, and those can be okay in moderation.

4. Limit calorie intake. Eat until satisfied, not full.

The basic truth is that if you consume more calories than you spend, you will gain weight.

A common mistake made even by people who eat "properly" is that they simply overeat: Too much of a good thing is still too much. So it is important to limit the calories you consume.

You don't have to count calories. Just learn to get in touch with your body and know when to stop eating.

When you follow the LSE rules, an interesting thing happens: Your body becomes proficient at utilizing calories rather than storing them. That in turn has two consequences: Your energy level increases; and you need to eat less to maintain that energy level, satisfy your appetite and stay satisfied.

It takes a little while for your brain to perceive the leptin signals that you have had enough to eat. The average person starting the **Flatten That Belly, Trim Those Thighs** eating plan takes 15-20 minutes to feel full.

The longer you follow the LSE rules, the shorter that time becomes because your body becomes very responsive to leptin.

So instead of eating till you feel full, stop eating when you feel **satisfied**. You'll know you are satisfied when you can honestly say this: **I *could* eat more, but I don't *need* to eat more.** That is the difference between eating enough and eating too much.

Another good starting point is to cut your portions by ¼. That means make your portions ¾ of the size you think you need or are used to.

Trust me; if you do that honestly, you will find you need much less food than you thought. And contrary to what you might think, you won't feel hungry anytime soon, because your body is becoming proficient at using the calories that you just consumed and at converting into energy calories stored as fat.

5. Finish eating at least three hours before bed.

Sleep time is an important fat-burning time.

You can burn a lot of fat in your sleep if you do things right.

Remember, three to four hours after you eat, the glycogen in your liver is depleted and you start using fat for metabolic functions.

So if you go to bed when you are in fat-burning mode, *all of your sleep time will be fat-burning time.* Granted, your metabolic rate is low when you sleep. Then again, you're getting six to eight hours of effortless fat burning.

Sleeping time is also an important healing time. It's when your body takes a break from many of its waking tasks, such as digestion, and turns all its attention to important healing and recovery functions. Don't distract your body from its repair work by making it digest food on the swing shift!

Some people are used to eating before bed and may find it hard to suddenly go without. The body has gotten used to a bad habit, and the brain is no longer perceiving the body's signals that it needs a break.

Again, just stick with it. Trust me. Not only will you get used to it, but you will realize how great it feels to go to sleep on an empty stomach.

Just don't overdo it. You don't want to go to bed more than six hours after eating. Between three to six hours is your target range.

6. Eat a nice-sized breakfast, a nice-sized lunch, and a small dinner.

If you stopped eating at least three hours before bed and slept seven to eight hours, you will have been fasting for about ten hours when you wake. Now is time to get your body going again.

A good breakfast with plenty of protein and (good) fat will allow you to start your day with energy and will ensure that you stay away from snacks and other temptations before lunch.

A good lunch likewise is important for it will keep you away from those familiar mid-afternoon energy crashes and cravings.

Many people give up waiting for dinner and give in to some junk food beforehand.

Proponents of "several small meals" will say, "Just have a healthy snack." However, my experience is that most people have a hard time thinking of anything healthy, much less preparing or eating it, when they are starving—which they will be by mid-afternoon if they had a light lunch.

In fact, I believe a "light" lunch is one of the biggest traps people fall into. With the best of intentions, you have a small salad with very little protein and very little fat, thinking, "That's a healthy lunch."

I predict that two hours later you feel like you are starving, fighting all kinds of cravings. And if (when) you do finally give in to the craving, you will blame yourself for lacking willpower. "Why do I have such a huge appetite?" Then, to make it worse, when dinner time comes, you're even hungrier *and* you've given up any hope of eating well. Next thing you know, it's time for bed.

Sound familiar?

One big challenge people encounter is late-night cravings. But guess what? The midnight munchies are not a necessary evil. No, these people are simply paying, late at night, for some crucial need of the body's that they neglected much, much earlier in the day.

If you have a nice breakfast and a nice lunch, cruising through the afternoon without food cravings and energy crashes will be easy. And when dinner time comes, you can have a light dinner. By the time you go to bed, your stomach is empty, and your body is ready to delve into those fat stores for seven to eight hours while you rest. Talk about sweet dreams!

7. Find your ideal macronutrient ratio.

Once you are eating all the right foods and adhering to the first six of the LSE rules, the final step to perfect nutrition is to find your **ideal macronutrient ratio**[1].

Although every human requires the same nutrients, the quantity of each macronutrient (protein, carbs, fat) is unique to each individual, influenced by both lifestyle and individual metabolism. That ratio also can change from meal to meal.

Most people do better with a high-protein breakfast and lunch, with less protein at dinner, which is also a smaller, lighter meal. This too might change from person to person.

Someone might do well on a high-protein diet but have to really watch carbs. This person's macronutrient ratio might be 40-30-30 (40 percent of the day's calories coming from protein, 30 percent from carbohydrates, 30 percent from fat).

Someone else might need more carbs but should be careful to limit protein and fat intake. This person's macronutrient ratio would be 30-50-20 (30 percent protein, 50 percent carbs, 20 percent fat).

This is an industry-standard presentation, but it's complicated to compute. The good news is that I have found a simpler—and more effective—way to identify your ideal macronutrient ratio: Gauge how you feel.

We in the modern world have "unlearned" this basic human instinct, but really all you need to do is to be mindful of your body's reactions. Observe how you feel after eating. If you're quiet and check in, you will "hear" the message it's trying to give you. Soon this effort becomes instinct, the way it was meant to be.

If you feel satisfied (not "stuffed") and full of energy, remain satisfied for several hours, and have no cravings between meals, what you ate was correct and in the proper ratio. Eating this way will give you optimal health and help you achieve your optimal weight.

Conversely, if you ate from the food chart but feel hungry right after eating; feel stuffed, heavy, or tired; have cravings; or get hungry in just a few hours, you need to adjust your ratio of macronutrients.

In my years of experience, I have found that most people have a good sense of their ideal macronutrient ratio. The problem starts when we get bombarded with so much conflicting information; it's easy to get out of touch with that basic instinct.

I begin with the assumption that you have some idea of your ideal macronutrient ratio. (If you don't, that's fine; the process still works. It'll just take a little more trial and error.) Here is what you do:

Imagine that you are going to a buffet. There you will find all of the foods that you like that are on the food chart. Your goal is to eat what you like **and** feel good afterward. What do you eat, and how much of it?

Whatever you think feels right is your starting point.

One person might say, "I can load up on protein and fat; so long as I don't eat a lot of carbs, I'll be fine." Another person might say, "I can eat a good amount of carbs, but if I eat too much protein and fat I'll feel heavy and bloated." Someone else might notice his plate has an equal balance of protein, carbs, and fat.

Now, for the next few days, plan and put together your meals this way.

Very quickly after eating mindfully, you will know if you were spot on. You feel satisfied and full of energy, stay satisfied for five to six hours till the next meal, and have no cravings. If that's the case, congratulations! You already "knew" your ideal macronutrient ratio.

If you don't feel quite right with your starting ratio, you will know that right away too. Use the following guidelines to identify your body's clues to "symptoms" and adjust accordingly.

---

[1] I learned this process while studying Metabolic Typing™ with William L. Wolcott, author of "The Metabolic Typing Diet"

Full, stuffed, heavy: You ate too much of one of the macronutrients--usually protein, but it might be carbs. Try cutting down on the suspect at the next meal. If the symptom persists, try cutting down on the other. Also use common-sense clues: If you ate plenty of carbs and only a small amount of protein, then carbs is the likely culprit. Start there.

Tired, sleepy: Again, too much of one of the macronutrients--usually carbs, but it can be protein. Again, cut down on the suspected macronutrient at the next meal and see how you feel. Again, rely on common sense: If you ate a good amount of protein and went light on carbs, most likely protein is the culprit.

Upset stomach or digestion problems: Usually too much fat. Again try cutting it down, and again use common sense. Of course, overeating anything can upset your stomach or intestines.

Not satisfied, still hungry; "full but still hungry": Not enough of one or more of the macronutrients--usually fat. Second most typical is protein.

Hungry too soon: Not enough of one or more macronutrients; it's usually fat that's deficient but could be any of the three.

Cravings: Too many carbs or not enough protein. Increase protein and/or decrease carbs, especially from starchy and moderately starchy foods.

Remember: *Your macronutrient ratio can change from meal to meal,* so do the same process for breakfast, lunch, and dinner. You may feel great by eating a high-protein breakfast but not so great if you do the same for dinner.

At first this process might seem difficult, but the work is a worthy process. Once you identify your ideal macronutrient ratio and how to detect its shifts, you will have mastered one of the most important elements of healthy eating. A too-tight waistline or a tell-tale scale should never again surprise you. You will always know if what you are eating is healthy and whether it will be fattening or will help you lose weight.

Eat this way and you will be on your way to a lifetime of optimal health and ideal weight.

The Leptin Sensitivity Enhancement Food Table

How to Use the LSE Food Table:

Because **all of your meals must be composed of protein, carbohydrate and fat**, every meal must include foods from the **Protein, Carbohydrates** and **Fat** groups. Items in the **Carbohydrates and Protein** group contain both protein and carbs. The listed spices not only taste great but also have anti-inflammatory properties and will help increase metabolism. Use them in every meal or as often as you can.

The Leptin Sensitivity Enhancement Food Table

Protein

Beef (lean)
Chicken
Canned chicken (in water)
Cottage cheese (low-fat)
Eggs
Ham
Hot dog (lean, uncured)
Pork (lean)
Sausage (lean)
Turkey
Seafood
 - Ahi tuna
 - Albacore tuna
(fresh or canned in water or olive oil)

- Calamari
- Catfish
- Cod
- Crab
- Flounder
- Freshwater bass
- Freshwater trout
- Mahi-mahi
- Salmon (best)
- Snapper
- Shrimp
- Tilapia
- Whitefish

Fat

Almond butter★★
Avocado
Avocado oil★★
Flax-seed oil
Healthy mayo★
Olive oil
Olive oil mayonnaise
Safflower oil (high-oleic only)★★
Sunflower oil (high-oleic only)★★
Healthy butter★

Carbohydrates and Protein

Beans (any kind)
Cheese (low-fat)
Garbanzo beans
Lentils
Manna From Heaven bread★★
Milk (organic, 1%, low-fat)
Nuts (also rich in good fats):
 - Almonds
 - Brazil nuts
 - Hazelnuts
 - Macadamia nuts
 - Pecans
 - Pine nuts
 - Pistachios
 - Walnuts
Protein bar (low-carb)
Protein shakes (low-carb)
Tofu
Veggie burgers (low-carb)
Yogurt (plain, low-fat)

Carbohydrates

LOW-STARCH VEGGIES
Artichoke
Asparagus
Arugula
Bell pepper
Bok choy
Broccoli
Brussels sprouts
Cabbage
Cauliflower
Celery
Chard
Collards
Cucumber
Eggplant
Green beans
Kale
Leeks
Lettuce (Romaine)
Mushrooms
Okra
Scallions
Spinach
Sprouts
Zucchini

WHOLE GRAINS & MODERATE STARCH VEGGIES
Buckwheat
Brown rice
Carrots
Kasha★★
Oats
Potato
Sprouted bread★★
Sprouted pasta★★
Squashes
Sweet potato
Whole-grain cereal
Wild rice★★
Yam

} Very little

LOW-FRUCTOSE FRUITS
Avocado
Olives

FRUITS
Apple
Banana
Berries
Cherries
Grapes
Grapefruit
Kiwi
Mango
Melons
Papaya
Peach
Pear
Pineapple
Pomegranate
Tomato

} OK in small amounts

Spices

Basil, Black Pepper, Cardamom, Chives, Cilantro, Cinnamon, Cloves, Cumin, Garlic, Ginger, Onion, Parsley, Rosemary, Thyme, Turmeric

★See recipe within "Some Cool and Easy Recipes" section.

★★ Go to eduardodias.com/resources for specialty items or anything that you can't easily find in your grocery store.

Tips for Success

Drink enough water.

Your body is mostly made of protein, fat and water, which must be replenished. So you must drink enough water. It might be the single most important element of our diet. Man can survive days, even weeks, without food; in certain conditions, Man couldn't survive even a day without water.

Water is the main component of hydrolysis, a chemical reaction that is part of the digestion of protein, starches and fats; it also is involved in energy production. And it's essential for weight loss.

The general daily guideline for most healthy adults is to drink 64 to 96 oz. (two to three liters or eight to 12 cups), a figure that can be widely influenced by climate conditions and activity level. It is not unusual for my clients to drink more than a gallon (128 oz.) on a summer day that includes a difficult workout.

Here is an additional guideline: Consider the color of your urine. Because the urinary system helps with elimination, the amount of water you intake will influence how much liquid you eliminate and how much water your body uses to eliminate metabolic byproducts. Dark urine probably means you're not drinking enough water. Your urine shouldn't be as clear as water but should be very light in color. If this is not the case, step up water consumption.

Some people have a hard time drinking water, saying it lacks flavor. If you feel this way, try herbal tea, iced or hot; sweeten with Stevia if desired. Most people can handle one daily cup of caffeinated tea; avoid more. Too much caffeine will overwork the thyroid and create all kinds of metabolic problems.[1]

Avoid drinking more than ½ cup of water (or any liquid) with a meal.

Although you should drink plenty of water throughout the day, avoid drinking too much when you eat.

One of two things will happen when you drink a lot of liquids with meals. One, the liquid will take up space in your stomach, giving you a false sense of satisfaction, causing your stomach to feel full. Soon that water will be absorbed and you will get hungry in fewer than five to six hours. Or, two, your stomach will expand to adjust to the higher volume you are consuming. This is often the cause of having a big belly. Sometimes people don't even have a lot fat around their bellies, but they have a big belly because their stomach has expanded to hold all the food and liquid they constantly ingest.

Further, digestion is a series of chemical reactions in your stomach and small intestine. Consumed food is combined with enzymes and broken down to be absorbed by the body. Introducing a lot of liquid into your stomach at the same time dilutes those enzymes and hinders digestion.

The rule is to drink no more than ½ cup of any liquid with a meal and wait one to two hours before drinking again. After that, drink up!

Water will get you through.

If you get enough protein, carbs, and fat, you should have no problem waiting five to six hours before your next meal. However, especially in the early days of this plan, your body might try to make you "think" you are hungry.

You shouldn't be.

Yes, your stomach is empty, but your body has plenty of stored fat for fuel.

However, you may be accustomed to the feeling of having something in your stomach all the time from

---

[1]   Later I cover the concept of personal "poisons"(pg. 14); then you can decide if you should eliminate caffeine altogether.

constant snacking. You might need help while you get used to being comfortable on an empty stomach.

Drinking extra water will help you through that. Every time you feel hunger pangs, drink a glass of water. You will be surprised how effective that is in killing those hunger pangs, and you will get the additional benefit of hydrating.

Use Stevia.

The Stevia plant, originally from Central and South America, is used for this extract, now widely available in the United States. To date, it is the only wholly natural sweetener known to have no negative side effects. If you need to sweeten anything, use Stevia; it leaves a very sweet taste but contains no sugar. Stay away from sugar, honey, and artificial sweeteners.

Stay fresh.

Always try to use fresh and organic ingredients when preparing meals.

Make sure to get adequate amounts of vitamins and minerals.

Vitamins and minerals are called micronutrients, but that doesn't mean they are unimportant. It means that compared to protein, carbs, and fat, you need very small amounts of them, but they are nonetheless absolutely essential to the chemical reactions in your body.

Theoretically, eating a balanced, plentiful diet should provide you with all the vitamins and minerals you need. Unfortunately, because of poor agricultural methods, our soils have become depleted, and today most fruits and vegetables don't contain the amount of nutrients they should. Our meats also tend to lack adequate amounts of key nutrients. Therefore you should supplement your diet with outside sources of nutrients in the form of a good-quality multivitamin supplement.

Be prepared!

One of the main reasons people fail on diets is because instead of having a planned, prepared meal, they eat whatever is available. Always have good food available at home, work, or wherever you go; the Eduardo's Super Soup[1] is great for that. Take time to plan and/or cook meals so you don't get caught short.

Have a "treat meal" once a week.

A treat meal lets you have anything that is not part of this plan--pizza, cheeseburger, chocolate, pie, cake, candy, soda--anything not on the food chart.

The reason for this is that *you must never feel deprived of the foods you like.*

If I were to tell you that you must never again eat anything that is not on the chart *for the rest of your life*, I would be asking you to fail.

And every time you strayed, you'd feel like you have no willpower. Honestly, I could not go on without pizza! I simply decide when I have it. And because I'm "allowed" to have it, it has lost its hold on me. I can't remember the last time I had a pizza, but if I ever feel like it, I know I will tell myself, "Let's wait until Saturday or Sunday."

It is much easier to say, "I will have it later," than, "I won't have it at all." If you know you will be eating that piece of chocolate or that slice of pie on Saturday, it's easier to say no to it when someone brings temptation into the office or when the waiter offers the dessert menu.

Of course, *when you have your treat meal, make sure you still follow as many of the LSE rules as you can.*

For example, you may have a starchy food and a dessert. Just make sure you don't stuff yourself with it; remember to get your protein and good fat with that meal; and wait five to six hours before you eat again. If you "break" one rule by overeating carbs, you can still follow the others. If you limit yourself to one broken rule once a week, you will be okay[2].

---

[1] See recipes. (pg. 20)
[2] See "What Is Your Poison?" (pg. 14) for exceptions.

Find sources of pleasure other than food and unhealthy stuff.

Remember the slogan "Just Say No"? The anti-drug people knew they had to provide something to "say yes" to.

If drugs is a social group's only source of pleasure, acceptance, activity, sense of belonging, even economic advancement (real or perceived), why would a member of that group refuse it? Kids need something new to fill the void created by saying "no," or they'll go back to their old ways.

The same thing goes for eating healthy and leading a healthy lifestyle. Many people turn to unhealthy eating because it is the only pleasure in their lives.

If you have a job you hate, people in your life who don't really bring you happiness or make you feel good, nothing that gives you pleasure, you may be turning to unhealthy eating for unhealthy reasons. And trying to control your eating when it is the only source of pleasure in your life won't work in the long run.

So I invite you to take a hard, honest look at your life. What do you enjoy? Do you love life? Do you at least like most of the things you spend your time on?

If you don't, I urge you to consider healthy and positive sources of pleasures--a hobby, a club of like-minded people. We are all unique, and the possibilities are endless, so *you can find your thing.* And it does not have to be food.

The good news is that doing healthy and positive things usually brings about an upward spiral and more healthy and positive things. The next thing you know, positive people and new pleasures will start showing up in your life. And suddenly those bad habits that seemed so hard to shake off won't even be an issue anymore.

What Is Your Poison?

Over the years I have come to discover that all of us have what I call our "poison." Your poison is that one or few things that you have to watch out for all the time, something that has a power over you beyond something you just like.

I compare it to an addiction. Actually, it *is* an addiction. For some, it's sugar in general or a specific such as soda or candy. For others it's starches, and again, it can be starches in general or a specific kind, such as breads. You might surrender totally to fatty, rich foods. You might overeat, binge eat, or eat emotionally. Different people have different poisons. Whatever your poison is, that's what you must look out for.

Your poison can wreak havoc in your goals.

You might be doing everything else right but *because of your poison* you can't lose weight, or get the body you want, or correct your health. Or you might be doing everything right until you give in to your poison, lose control, and lose all that ground.

Over the years as a personal trainer, I've helped hundreds of people to lose weight. I have great success stories of people who lost hundreds of pounds and completely changed their lives.

Of course, I also have stories that I consider learning experiences for me. Two heartbreaking stories illustrate what a poison can do.

Mary's Story

The first case is about a wonderful woman; let's call her Mary. Mary was about 150 pounds overweight and came to me determined to lose weight.

I love it when someone walks into the gym with that kind of determination, because I know that person is up for a great and rewarding journey. It's beautiful to see someone's life change like that. And I had a strong feeling that Mary would be one of those.

Mary knew exactly what her "problems" were. (I hadn't discovered the concept of poisons back then.) Her problems were sugar and starches. Her entire life she had been controlled by overeating, but her overeating was deeply linked to eating sweets and starchy foods.

When she came to me she already had quit eating *anything* sweet or starchy. No sodas, no bread, no candy. Nothing. Ever. Because, she said, the minute she ate one little candy bar or drank one soda it was like a monster awoke inside of her and that monster couldn't be satisfied. It always wanted more and more. So she finally swore off those.

With this insight, we figured out that the right kind of diet for Mary was a high-protein diet with lots of vegetables and very little, if any, fruits.

With our workouts and her new eating plan, Mary started losing a safe, healthy average of 10 pounds per month! She was new woman. She was positive, optimistic, talking about finding her dream guy, wearing a bikini, going to her high school reunion, and blowing people away. It was amazing!

In one year she lost more than 100 pounds. I figured that in a few months Mary would be at her ideal weight.

On her one-year anniversary of swearing off her poisons, Mary decided to treat herself to a cupcake. ONE CUPCAKE.

Well, the woman who walked into the gym on that Monday was not the Mary I had seen on Friday. She was depressed to have given in to "temptation." She was pessimistic about being able to resist again. She kept talking about how her entire life she had been a heavy girl--completely ignoring the fact that she was on her way to being one of my biggest success stories.

From that day on, every time Mary came to work out she had an excuse for why she had eaten badly the day before, how her therapist was trying to work with her to get her to stop, why she had just been kidding herself for the entire year that she was doing good.

I was literally talking to a different woman. She was on her way to failure, and nothing I said or did seemed to help. She stopped losing weight and started to miss workouts. Ultimately she dropped out all together.

ONE CUPCAKE changed her eating habits, her entire psyche, her life.

Cathy's Story

Here's another story. Let's call this client Cathy. Cathy was a very pretty, very big girl. She was over 6 feet tall and about 100 pounds overweight.

She told me she had been working out by herself for one month doing cardio but hadn't lost a pound.

I've had countless people come to me over the years with a similar situation. I knew exactly what to do to get her to lose weight. I needed to get her on a good eating program and start her on strength training, because cardio alone was not doing the trick.

Somehow, however, Cathy was not responding to our strategy.

I knew she was doing the right thing as far as the workouts because she was with me. So I figured she must have been doing something wrong as far as the eating. I had her start writing down everything she ate. Everything. From her meals to every glass of water.

I was surprised when Cathy brought me food journals that showed perfect meals. I couldn't believe it. If that food journal was true, she was one of the most diligent healthy eaters I had ever seen; even on the weekends she was perfect. Yet she couldn't lose the weight. I couldn't understand it.

One day in conversation with a mutual friend I happened to learn Cathy's secret: She was a heavy drinker. She went out on dates almost every night. Because she was so big, she could handle large amounts of alcohol—and she drank *a lot*.

It all made sense then; alcohol was her poison. It didn't matter how well she was eating; the alcohol was not only bringing a lot of calories into her diet, but it was also wreaking havoc on her system, completely neutralizing any effort she made to balance her metabolism.

Even though she was eating perfectly otherwise, the alcohol didn't allow her to lose weight. And she knew it. She hired me hoping I could make her lose weight in spite of her drinking. When I asked her about it, she denied it. Soon after, she dropped out of training.

Those two stories illustrate perfectly what your poison can do to you. We *all* have our poisons; it's just that, for some, the poison has a stronger hold.

You probably already know your poison. And you are probably hoping I'm not talking about that one. Or those two. Or three.

Well, yes, I am, and you know it. You've probably already skipped ahead to skim the list.

If you honestly don't know you poison, think about the foods you crave that have a particularly strong hold on you. Maybe it is as bad as sugar was for Mary. Could one taste unleash a monster that can't be satiated? Is there one thing you think you can't live without, despite its effects, like alcohol was for Cathy?

If you have struggled with weight for a while, if you have struggled with bad eating habits—I'd hazard a guess that 90 percent of the time, if you have a chronic health issue, your poison is *the* cause.

And you must quit it. Period.

The greater the hold your poison has on you, the more important and urgent it is that you conquer it.

And once you do, *that alone will lead you to success.*

A lot of people don't take control over their poison because they think, "What's the use? I'm never going to have the body I want anyway." Or, "I'll never straighten up my health anyway, so I might as well enjoy my poison."

Don't think like that. Take control over your poison and you will succeed.

In fact, most of the time, taking control of your poison doesn't necessarily mean you can't ever have it. Of course, the greater the hold, the more likely it is that you will have to swear it off for good. That's what Mary's case proved.

Most people, however, don't have to stay away from their poisons 100 percent of the time. The keys are total awareness, an ability to recognize and regulate "once in a while," and the self-control for "just a little bit."

Always be careful, because a poison can creep up on you. They are tricky. You think you're in control, and meanwhile it is slowly making its way back into your life.

Of all the poisons I have encountered, I have found that alcohol and sugar are the two that generally require quitting rather than cutting back.

It sounds harder than it is. When you do get rid of a poison and get it out of your system, it no longer has that power over you, and it becomes easier to say no.

Of course, that can also be dangerous as well. Like Mary, you might decide one day to have a little bit of your poison, not because you *need* to it anymore, but because once it no longer has any power over you (or so you think), you can enjoy it like everyone else.

That is the biggest mistake you can make.

Your poison can take over your life with a vengeance, just as it did in Mary's case, and not let go. Ever.

If you feel this could be you, don't risk it. Stay away from your poison completely. Again, it is not so hard once you eliminate the habit. And the rewards are tremendous.

Here is a list of the most common poisons. Which is yours?

> Starchy foods (breads, pasta, white rice anything made with white flour)
> Pastries, donuts, pies, cakes
> Sugar (anything sweet)
> Sodas
> Candy
> Fatty foods, anything creamy, rich, or full of butter
> Overeating
> Binge eating
> Constant eating (eating all the time)
> Emotional eating (eating for comfort when sick, sad, angry, happy, etc.)
> Chocolate
> Coffee or caffeine
> Dairy (If you crave cheese, ice cream, or even plain milk, dairy may be your poison; this can create an imbalance in your endocrine system that will result in weight gain and have other negative consequences to your health.)
> Ice cream
> Alcohol
> Salty Foods

I would love to hear if you think your poison is not on this list. Tell me your story. What had a hold of you? How were you able to defeat it? And if you haven't, maybe I can help. Contact me via my website: www.eduardodias.com/contact.

Troubleshooting

This plan works; there is no question. For years my clients have followed it and arrived at this wonderful place where eating is effortless and pleasurable and keeps them healthy and at their ideal weight.

If you find that the plan is not working, or if it works for a while and then seems to stop, the first thing you should do is to go back and reread the plan. I would bet you'll find you have misremembered one or more of the rules and are not following them correctly.

Here are some common mistakes that can hinder efforts or make it appear as if the plan is not working:

Following the plan halfway, or following some rules but not others.

Some people may decide some rules are not as important or are too hard to follow. The truth is you will never know if something works until you have given it a full shot. If you have decided to follow this plan, follow it 100 percent.

At the very least, if it doesn't work, you'll know it's not your fault, right?

But I know this works.

It has *never* failed if people followed it 100 percent. So give it a complete try; follow all the principles; and work out whatever issues you need to work out.

Straying off the plan too much.

We are all human, and we can't be perfect all the time. I include the treat meal once a week so that you never feel deprived, and that makes it easier to stick with the plan. In reality, however, we all have little slips here and there aside from the treat meal.

Try to stick with the plan as much as you can. Especially in the beginning. *Discipline is a matter of habit.* And if you get in the habit of being loose with your eating, it will have a big impact—a big, negative impact.

I've had people having a hard time losing weight who told me they were following the diet pretty well. Yet when I had them write down everything they ate, all sorts of "little things" would show up, like a "small" piece of pie right after a meal as a reward for behaving. Or "just a few" potato chips between meals.

If weight loss is your goal, I suggest that you go 100 percent on the plan until you have reached your optimum weight. Then you can be a little more lenient and see how much your body can tolerate. But be careful: If discipline is a matter of habit, and you start being looser and looser, next thing you know you may get completely get off the track.

Getting hungry because you are not drinking enough water.

Not drinking enough water is one of the most common reasons why people get hungry between meals. In fact they are not hungry at all; they are just thirsty.

Water not only plays a role in the metabolism of fat into energy but also will keep you from getting that "empty stomach feeling."

This happens to me all the time: Two or three hours after a meal, I feel what I first think is hunger. But because I've been doing this long enough, I immediately realize that the problem is I have forgotten to drink water. I'm thirsty, not hungry.

So at the first sign of hunger, ask yourself: "Have I been drinking water since my last meal?" Drink a glass of water, and you may be surprised that the hunger disappears!

Getting hungry because you didn't get enough fat.

We have been so conditioned to fear fat that most people can only conceive of a healthy meal as being a low-fat meal. One consequence of the low-fat meal is that you'll get hungry again very soon.

In my plan, you should not be afraid of fat so long as you eat the right kind (the ones on the food table). In fact, you should eat plenty of those.

I've also seen this over and over: Someone tells me they are having a hard time waiting five to six hours between meals. When I have them write down what they're eating, I see these "fear of fat" meals. They add some olive oil but just a dash, or they have 1/8 of an avocado.

I wish I could tattoo it on your hands to look at again and again. This low-fat conditioning is one of the worst things we've immersed ourselves in. Please don't be afraid of fat. *So long as you are eating the right fats, fat is good.*

Eating too much saturated fat from dairy, red meat and pork.

Now that I just taunted you about how good fat is, I have to warn you again about the wrong kind of fat.

When people hear me saying that fat is okay, many say, "Oh, great, so I can eat any fat I want." That's not true either.

Saturated fat is very fattening. And it can sneak up on you.

Any fat is loaded with calories; just a few grams of saturated fat will add quite a few calories to your meals, calories that your body will easily convert into fat around your stomach and thighs.

When eating foods such as dairy, always choose the low-fat varieties; full-fat dairy is loaded with saturated fat. The same is true for red meat and pork; even leaner cuts of red meat and pork have quite a bit of saturated fat, so limit these. On my sample menus, red meat and pork show up once or twice a week. Most protein should come from chicken and fish.

Eating too much.

This plan will help your body become proficient at utilizing the calories you eat rather than storing them. One of the consequences is that you will need to eat less. The problem is some people are used to overeating and neglect to adjust the amount even when they start eating right.

On this plan, even if you overeat, you will most likely lose weight. But overeating may make the difference between achieving your ideal weight and being a few pounds over.

Some of my clients have a hard time shedding the last five to ten pounds. Those final pounds usually come off by being very diligent with eating **and** cutting down on portions by ¼.

Remember: *Eat until you are satisfied not until you are full.* You will be surprised at how little you need to be satisfied when you follow this plan.

Overeating on the weekend.

This falls into the category of overeating, but it's a special case. Some people are perfect during the week, but when the weekend comes they don't just cheat; they cheat the entire time, eating entirely too much. That can not only add quite a few pounds, but also it can hinder your ability to eat less on the other days.

Here is a cycle I have seen: Person tries to be "good" during the week. On the weekend, they let go and eat as much as they like of whatever they want. That alone makes them gain a little weight. On Monday they again try to control their eating, but for some reason they find it a little harder to go from no discipline to 100 percent discipline. But they keep at it throughout the week, getting more and more diligent until Friday comes around and they are having an easy time being perfect. Great!

But then the weekend comes, and the cycle starts again.

The solution is: *Never give in to the temptation of overeating.* Overeating can be a "sneaky little monster" that will creep up on you. Next thing you know, you are overeating all the time and eating everything in front of you. At your treat meal, allow yourself to eat foods not on the plan but never allow yourself to overeat.

Not giving yourself enough time to get used to eating every five to six hours; giving up too soon.

Many people are unaccustomed to eating nothing between meals. They have been snacking or munching for so long that having nothing besides water or tea between meals can be hard to get used to.

If you are one of those, just *believe that you can*.

Unless you have a metabolic problem, you can and should get used to going five to six hours without eating anything. So stick with it.

I've had "chronic snackers" look at me like I was asking them swallow fire when I tell them not to snack. Yet not only have they been able to do it, but that act alone helped each one lose an amazing amount of weight.

You can do it. Just stick with it. Remember, drinking water will help.

If you suspect you may have a metabolic problem, consult your doctor, but 90 percent of the time, it is simply a matter of creating a new habit.

Eating too much at dinner or too close to bedtime.

In my sample menus, dinners are light. It is really important to observe the rule about finishing eating three hours before going to bed *and* making your dinner a light one.

Many people are used to having a big dinner and going to bed shortly after. Nevertheless, you must adapt to your lifestyle.

If you absolutely cannot arrange it so that you finish eating at least three hours before bed, make your dinner even lighter. The closer to bedtime, the less you should eat.

Not having a good lunch and then losing control at night.

As much as I tell people to watch for it, this is one thing I catch people doing over and over. I think it's because of the same social conditioning that tells people to fear fat.

At lunch you eat light and think you're doing well: "I'm behaving by eating my little salad with a tiny piece of skinless chicken and low-fat dressing." Willpower is high, and you feel great about yourself.

But by dinnertime you are ravenous and cannot control yourself. You blame yourself for lack of will-power. You might even overeat or eat badly to punish yourself. Who is that helping?

Yet if you are having problems at night, 90 percent of the time the sole reason is that you didn't have a substantial lunch with enough fat, protein and carbs.

Remember: A good lunch will keep you good for dinner.

Carb addiction

Sugar addiction is so serious it deserves to be mentioned again. If you are addicted to sugar, if sugar is your poison, most likely you will have to stay away from it forever.

In the body, starchy carbs convert to sugar very fast, so you'll probably have to stay away from those too. Unfortunately, there is no way around it. Telling a sugar addict that he can have some sugar and high starchy carbs and still control his diet is like telling an alcoholic that she can have a drink every now and then and still control her alcoholism. It can't be done.

Again, though, the good news is that if you do stay away, the benefit is a lifetime of health and ideal weight. Isn't that an acceptable tradeoff?

Some Delicious and Simple Recipes

Here are a few quick-to-prepare items that also appear in the sample menus. Having healthy options that are ready in advance or can be prepared quickly on the spot is one of the keys to success. Having go-to foods will make it easier to stay on track when you are short on time or just too hungry to prepare a full meal.

I hope that eventually you will try all of these recipes, but I strongly suggest that you begin with Eduardo's Super Soup. This has become one of the most popular elements of my food plan with my clients. They came up with the name, and it really is a "super" food. It's high in fiber, has everything you need (carbs, protein and fat) and it's very satisfying.

It's super-fast to prepare a whole batch. Put it in the fridge for up to a week; just warm it up when you're ready to eat.

Over the years, this soup has virtually guaranteed that my successful clients stay on track with their eating.

Once you have it available, you will be amazed at how many times you'll say, "I wish I had something to eat right now that's tasty, fast and healthy. Wait a minute--I do!"

It is the perfect lunch to take to work or school.

Come to think of it, it's also perfect for dinner after a long work day.

Actually, there is nothing wrong with having it for breakfast if you want.

It is a fast meal, but it is not a "meal substitute"; it is a meal in itself. Enjoy this and go about your day.

EDUARDO'S SUPER SOUP

3 lbs. of vegetables*, chopped

2 lbs. chicken (ground, diced or shredded)   3 tsp. basil

1 tsp. MSG-free seasoned salt (optional)   1-2 Tbs. olive oil, separated

1 liter of low-sodium chicken broth

1. Boil chicken 5-10 minutes in chicken broth with basil and (optional) seasoned salt.

2. Add vegetables and boil everything for an additional 10-15 minutes.

3. Let cool and refrigerate.

4. Add 1-2 tablespoons of olive oil when you heat it up to eat.

*Any of the following: spinach, asparagus, carrot, green beans, onion, cauliflower, broccoli, Brussels sprouts, celery, artichoke, bell pepper, mushrooms, sprouts (any kind).

EDUARDO'S "BERRY AWESOME" SHAKE

1 scoop of casein protein powder*

1 cup milk, 1% low-fat milk or almond milk

1/2 cup berries (blueberries, raspberries, blackberries, strawberries or a mix of these)

Add it all in a blender and blend it.

* At the time of this writing, whey protein is the most popular protein around. Whey is great for a post workout meal, but for regular meals whey gets absorbed too quickly by your body, which means you will get hungry soon. Casein protein takes longer to be absorbed and will keep you satisfied for longer, so it's the one I recommend for regular meals.

EDUARDO'S HEALTHY BUTTER

This is the perfect substitute for butter or margarine. It has one quarter of the saturated fat of butter. Instead, we add more monounsaturated fat from avocado oil, high-oleic sunflower or high-oleic safflower oil. It is also much softer than butter, so it's spreadable right out of the fridge.

1/2 cup butter (usually one stick)

1 1/2 cup avocado oil, high-oleic sunflower oil or high-oleic safflower oil

In a 2-cup container, add butter (make sure it's soft) with oil and mix with a mixer, wire whisk or hand blender (a mixer or hand blender will make it more homogeneous).

Refrigerate.

Tip: Only remove from fridge right before you use it, or it'll be too soft. For a harder consistency (but less of the good fats), use 1 cup of butter and 1 cup of oil.

EDUARDO'S HEALTHY MAYO*

2 omega-3 egg yolks

1 teaspoon Dijon mustard

1/8 teaspoon of sea salt

1/2 cup high-oleic sunflower oil, high-oleic safflower oil or avocado oil

1 Tbs. lemon juice or white wine vinegar

1. In a bowl or food processor add Dijon mustard, egg yolks, salt and lemon juice/vinegar. Mix with electric mixer or in a food processor.

2. Slowly add the oil as you continue mixing or running the food processor. Add the oil slowly or it won't mix correctly and the mayo will be too runny.

3. Refrigerate for up to one week. (Double or triple the ingredients if you think you will use the mayo within one week.)

* Go on my website (www.eduardodias.com) for a video of me showing how to make Eduardo's healthy mayo.

AVOCADO SPREAD, FULL VERSION

1 avocado, medium

1/4 cup onion, chopped

1 clove garlic, minced

1/4 cup tomato, chopped

1/4 cup cilantro, chopped

1 Tbs. lime juice

1/8 tsp. chili powder

1/8 tsp. sea salt

1. Place all the ingredients in a medium size bowl and smash together with a fork.

2. Refrigerate and use within 48 hours.

QUICK AVOCADO SPREAD

1 medium avocado

1/8 teaspoon seasoned salt, MSG-free

1. Smash the avocado in a small bowl, mixing in the seasoned salt.

2. Refrigerate and use within 48 hours.

CHICKEN AND AVOCADO SPREAD

1 can of chicken (10 oz.)

1 avocado, medium

1/8 teaspoon seasoned salt, MSG-free

1. Smash the avocado in a small bowl, mixing in seasoned salt.

2. Mix in the chicken.

3. Refrigerate and use within in 48 hours.

CHICKEN SPREAD WITH EDUARDO'S HEALTHY MAYO

1 can chicken (10-12 oz.)

1-2 Tbs. Eduardo's Healthy Mayo OR olive oil mayonnaise

1. Mix all the ingredients in a bowl with a fork.

2. Refrigerate and eat within 48 hours.

TUNA SPREAD WITH EDUARDO'S HEALTHY MAYO

1 can tuna (5 oz.)

1/2 - 1 Tbs. Eduardo's Healthy Mayo OR olive oil mayonnaise

1. Mix all the ingredients in a bowl with a fork.

2. Refrigerate and eat within 48 hours.

SALMON PATÉ

7oz. salmon, fresh or canned

3 oz. nonfat or low-fat cream cheese

1/2 tablespoon dill

If using fresh salmon, mix all ingredients in a food processor.

If using canned salmon, drain salmon completely and then mix all ingredients in a

bowl with a fork.

Sample Menus

I'm going to give you three weeks' worth of menus according to the **Flatten That Belly, Trim Those Thighs** eating plan.

My goal is not to make you eat these 63 meals and nothing else. You could just rotate these menus and be fine. But ideally you will look at these menus and use them as a starting point to put together your own meals and weekly menus.

The main goal is for you to be able to see how we put together meals using the LSE rules: how to put together meals with protein, carbs, and fat from the allowed food table; how to make those meals low in carbs and saturated fat but still satisfying; how to put together a nice-sized breakfast, a nice-sized lunch, and a small dinner, etc. This way you can customize and put together meals according to your own taste.

Many of my clients do follow these menus for the first three weeks. It allows them to try everything and figure out what they like or dislike and what needs adjustment. After that, a client might experiment, using some of my suggested meals, some with modifications, and some completely new and different meals--all according to the LSE rules.

You will notice that I'm giving you options on the portions. That's because some people need to eat more than others. Also, according to your ideal macronutrient ratio, you might need bigger portions of different items. For example, you might need 6 oz of protein but a very small portion of carbs. Or you might need a larger portion of carbs and just 4 oz. of protein. You will figure that out as you follow the instructions in the "Find Your Macronutrient Ratio" section.

Most people will not be in the upper range of portion size. For example, 1 cup of garbanzo beans, 5 oz. of asparagus and 8 oz of meat is a pretty big meal suitable for more active people who need more calories. Most people don't need to eat that much and will have a problem if they do.

The more sedentary you are, the less you should eat. I suggest you start with the smallest suggested portions and go from there, especially if you are trying to lose weight. You may be surprised that, once your body adjusts to this way of eating, you will be satisfied with the smaller portions.

I strongly suggest that you buy a food scale. Although ultimately you will be able to size your portions just by looking, you will need to learn what 6 oz. of chicken breast or spinach looks like. I use my food scale all the time--just makes things easier.

Although I'm not including the Eduardo's Super Soup on the menus, I strongly recommend that you make and refrigerate it. I guarantee that, in the course of these three weeks, you will need a quick, healthy meal. Soup to the rescue! And of course you can substitute the soup for any scheduled meal that does not appeal to you.

WEEK 1 SAMPLE MENU

MONDAY

Breakfast:
- 1 cup 1% low-fat milk or almond milk
- 1 medium banana
- 1-3 scrambled eggs with 1 Tbs. of flax-seed oil, or cooked in olive oil, high-oleic (high-heat) sunflower oil, high-oleic (high-heat) safflower oil or avocado oil

Lunch:
- Chicken or turkey burger with low-fat cheese on sprouted-grain bread or bun
- Small salad (Romaine lettuce, shredded carrots, cucumber, tomatoes) with olive oil or low-fat dressing with 1 Tbs. of flax-seed oil

Dinner:
- Salad: 2-6 oz. chicken breast, spinach, tomatoes, cucumbers, carrots, garbanzo beans (or choice of beans) with olive oil or low-fat dressing with 1 Tbs. of flax-seed oil

TUESDAY

Breakfast:
- ¾-1 cup whole-grain cereal* with 1% low-fat milk or almond milk
- 3-8 oz. turkey sausage cooked with olive oil, high-oleic (high-heat)

sunflower oil, high-oleic (high-heat) safflower oil or avocado oil

Lunch:
- 1 cup (3.5 oz.) green beans sautéed with olive oil
- 3-8 oz. lean pork chops
- ¼-½ cup wild rice

Dinner:
- 3-5 oz. steamed vegetable mix: (cauliflower, broccoli, carrots, pearl onions) with olive oil
- 2-6 oz. broiled salmon

WEDNESDAY

Breakfast:
- Berry awesome shake with blueberries
- ½-1 medium avocado

Lunch:
- Chicken breast sandwich on sprouted-grain bread or bun with low-fat cheese and healthy mayo or olive oil mayonnaise
- ½-1 cup fruit salad (or any fruit from the food table)

Dinner:
- 1-2 slices sprouted-grain toast with avocado spread
- ¼-1 cup low-fat cottage cheese

THURSDAY

Breakfast:
- ½-1 cup oatmeal
- 1-3 scrambled eggs with 1 Tbs. of flax-seed oil, or cooked in olive oil, high-oleic (high-heat) sunflower oil, high-oleic (high-heat) safflower oil or avocado oil

Lunch:
- Asparagus (5-8 spears/3-5 oz.) sautéed with olive oil
- ½-1 cup garbanzo beans (or choice of beans)
- 3-8 oz. salmon

Dinner:
- Small sandwich with lean ham or sliced turkey and low-fat cheese on sprouted-grain bread with healthy mayo or olive oil mayonnaise

FRIDAY

Breakfast:
- Smoked salmon omelet: 2-3 eggs, 2-4 oz. smoked salmon
- 1-1½ cup (3-5 oz.) strawberries

Lunch:
- Tuna spread sandwich on sprouted -grain bread

SATURDAY

Breakfast:
- 1-2 Whole-grain pancakes
- 1-3 scrambled eggs with 1 Tbs. of flax-seed oil, or cooked in olive oil, high-oleic (high-heat) sunflower oil, high-oleic (high-heat) safflower oil or avocado oil
- 3-8 oz. chicken or turkey breakfast sausage

Lunch:
- Lean, uncured hot dogs on sprouted-grain bun** with healthy mayo or mustard

Dinner:
- Pizza: Sprouted-grain pizza crust**, low-sodium tomato sauce, low-fat mozzarella cheese and any of the following: lean ham, ground chicken or turkey with Italian seasoning, turkey bacon,

olives, onions, green peppers, mushrooms, garlic, tomatoes

SUNDAY

Breakfast:
- 1-3 scrambled eggs with 1 Tbs. of flax-seed oil, or cooked in olive oil, high-oleic (high-heat) sunflower oil, high-oleic (high-heat) safflower oil or avocado oil
- Small portion of hash browns or potatoes. Cooked with healthy butter or olive oil
- 2-4 oz. Turkey bacon

Lunch:
- Burrito: wild rice, pinto beans, low-fat cheese, avocados, shredded chicken with Mexican seasoning** on a sprouted-grain tortilla**

Dinner:
- Tuna wrap: 1 can of tuna in olive oil, lettuce, chopped tomatoes, avocado, on a sprouted-grain tortilla**

- Small salad (Romaine lettuce, shredded carrots, cucumber, tomatoes) with olive oil or low-fat dressing with 1 Tbs. of flax-seed oil

Dinner:
- ½-1 cup low-fat plain yogurt with ½ cup diced strawberries; sweeten with Stevia if needed
- ¼-½ medium avocado

*Suggested whole-grain cereals: Fiber One, All Bran, Total, Cheerios. Fiber One and All Bran are my favorites because of the high fiber content.

** Go to www.eduardodias.com/resources for specialty items or anything that you can't find easily in your grocery store.

27

WEEK 2 SAMPLE MENU

MONDAY

Breakfast:
- Berry awesome shake with strawberries
- ½–1 medium avocado

Lunch:
- Chicken avocado spread sandwich on sprouted-grain bread
- Small salad (Romaine lettuce, shredded carrots, cucumber, tomatoes) with olive oil or low-fat dressing with 1 Tbs. of flax-seed oil

Dinner:
- Smoothie: 1 cup 1% low-fat milk or almond milk, ½ cup frozen mixed berries
- ¼–½ cup almonds

TUESDAY

Breakfast:
- Omelet: 2-3 eggs, spinach, low-fat cheese, turkey bacon
- 1-2 slices sprouted-grain toast with healthy butter

Lunch:
- 3–8 oz. Shrimp sautéed with olive oil, garlic and black pepper
- ¼–½ cup wild rice

- ¼ –½ cup black beans (or choice of beans)

Dinner:
- 3–5 oz. steamed vegetable mix (broccoli, green beans, bell peppers, carrots) with olive oil
- 2-6 oz. grilled chicken breast

WEDNESDAY

Breakfast:
- ¼–1 cup low-fat cottage cheese with one Tbs. of flax-seed oil
- ½–1 medium apple
- 1-2 slices sprouted-grain toast with healthy butter

Lunch:
- Tuna spread sandwich on sprouted-grain bread
- ½–1 cup fruit salad (or any fruit from the food table)

Dinner:
- Salad: 2-6 oz. grilled salmon, Romaine lettuce, tomatoes, cucumbers, carrots, garbanzo beans (or choice of beans) with olive oil or low-fat dressing with 1 Tbs. of flax-seed oil

THURSDAY

Breakfast:
- 1-3 hard-boiled eggs
- ½–1 cup whole-grain cereal* with 1% low-fat milk or almond milk
- ½–1 medium avocado

Lunch:
- 1-2 chicken or turkey burger patty
- ¼–½ cup pinto beans (or choice of beans)
- ¼–½ cup carrots sautéed with olive oil

Dinner:
- ½–1 cup low-fat plain yogurt with 1-2 Tbs. blueberries; sweeten with Stevia if needed
- ¼–½ medium avocado

FRIDAY

Breakfast:
- ½–1 cup oatmeal
- 1-2 gourmet chicken sausages**
- ½–1 medium avocado

SATURDAY

Breakfast:
- 1-3 scrambled eggs with 1 Tbs. of flax-seed oil or cooked with olive oil, high-oleic (high-heat) sunflower oil, high-oleic (high-heat) safflower oil or avocado oil
- Small portion of hash browns or country potatoes cooked with healthy butter or olive oil
- 3–6 oz. Lean pork chops

Lunch:
- **Lean** hamburger (or chicken or turkey burger) with low-fat cheese on a sprouted-grain bread or bun
- Small salad (Romaine lettuce, shredded carrots, cucumber, tomatoes) with olive oil or low-fat dressing with 1 Tbs. of flax-seed oil

SUNDAY

Breakfast:
- Healthy Eggs Benedict: Sprouted-grain English muffin** with healthy butter, Canadian bacon, eggs cooked with olive oil, high-oleic (high-heat) sunflower oil, high-oleic (high-heat) safflower oil or avocado oil

Lunch:
- Grilled ham and cheese sandwich: 3-6 oz. lean ham, low-fat cheese on sprouted-grain bread grilled with healthy butter
- ½–1 cup fruit salad (or any fruit from the food table)

Dinner:
- Shrimp wrap: 2-6 oz. baby shrimp, lettuce, tomatoes, and avocado on a sprouted-grain tortilla**

Lunch:
- 3–8 oz. grilled salmon
- 1 cup (3 oz.) spinach sautéed with olive oil
- ½–1 cup green peas

Dinner:
- ½–1 sprouted-grain English muffin** with salmon paté

Dinner:
- Gnocchi (small portion) with low-sodium tomato sauce, 2-6 oz. ground chicken or turkey, olive oil and Italian seasoning

*Suggested whole-grain cereals: Fiber One, All Bran, Total, Cheerios. Fiber One and All Bran are my favorites because of the high fiber content.

** Go to www.eduardodias.com/resources for specialty items or anything that you can't find easily in your grocery store.

28

WEEK 3 SAMPLE MENU

MONDAY

Breakfast:
- Frittata: 1-3 eggs, mushrooms, spinach and tomatoes cooked with olive oil, high-oleic (high-heat) sunflower oil, high-oleic (high-heat) safflower oil or avocado oil
- ½-1 cup whole-grain cereal* with 1% low-fat milk or almond milk

Lunch:
- 3-8 oz. seared ahi tuna
- Asparagus (5-8 spears/3-5 oz.) sautéed with olive oil
- ¼-½ cup wild rice

Dinner:
- ¼-1 cup low-fat cottage cheese with one Tbs. of flax-seed oil
- ¼-1 cup cashews (or any nuts from the table)

TUESDAY

Breakfast:
- ¼-1 cup low-fat cottage cheese with one Tbs. of flax-seed oil
- 1 medium pear
- 1-2 slices sprouted-grain toast with healthy butter

Lunch:
- Chicken breast sandwich on sprouted-grain bread or bun with low-fat cheese and healthy mayo or olive oil mayonnaise
- Small salad (Romaine lettuce, shredded carrots, cucumber, tomatoes) with olive oil or low-fat dressing with 1 Tbs. of flax-seed oil

Dinner:
- Greek salad: Romaine lettuce, tomatoes, cucumber, red onions, garbanzo beans, black olives and ¼-½ cup of feta cheese with olive oil

WEDNESDAY

Breakfast:
- Berry Awesome Shake with mixed berries
- ½-1 medium avocado

Lunch:
- 1-2 chicken or turkey burger patty
- 1 cup (3 oz.) cauliflower with low-fat cheese
- ½-1 medium avocado

Dinner:
- 3-5 oz. steamed vegetables (asparagus, green beans, bell peppers, celery) with olive oil
- 2-6 oz. grilled freshwater trout (or any fish from the food table)

THURSDAY

Breakfast:
- 1-2 gourmet chicken sausages**
- ½-1 cup oatmeal
- ½-1 medium avocado

Lunch:
- 3-8 oz. grilled salmon
- ¼-1 cup garbanzo beans (or choice of beans)
- Small salad (Romaine lettuce, shredded carrots, cucumber, tomatoes) with olive oil or low-fat dressing with 1 Tbs. of flax-seed oil

Dinner:
- Smoothie: 1 cup 1% low-fat milk or almond milk, ½ cup frozen strawberries
- ¼-½ cup low-fat cottage cheese
- ½-1 medium avocado

FRIDAY

Breakfast:
- Turkey and low-fat cheese omelet: 2-3 eggs, 2-4 oz. turkey and low-fat cheese
- Small serving of hash browns or country potatoes cooked with healthy butter or olive oil

Lunch:
- Tuna spread sandwich on sprouted-grain bread
- ½-1 cup fruit salad (or any fruit from the food table)

Dinner:
- ½-1 cup fruit salad (or any fruit from the food table)
- ½-1 cup plain yogurt; sweeten with Stevia
- ¼-½ cup macadamia nuts (or any nuts from the table)

SATURDAY

Breakfast:
- Breakfast burrito: 1- 2 eggs, 3-6 oz. ground chicken or turkey with Mexican seasoning**, diced potatoes cooked with olive oil, high-oleic (high-heat) sunflower oil, high-oleic (high-heat) safflower oil or avocado oil and low-fat cheese on a sprouted-grain tortilla**

Lunch:
- 3-8 oz. grilled, lean steak
- Small baked potato with low-fat sour cream and healthy butter
- 3-5 oz. grilled vegetable mix: bell peppers, zucchini, mushrooms

SUNDAY

Dinner:
- Turkey sandwich: 2-4 oz. turkey on sprouted-grain bread with low-fat cheese and healthy mayo or olive oil mayonnaise

Breakfast:
- French toast made with sprouted-grain bread
- Frittata: 2-3 scrambled eggs with low-fat cheese and 2-4 oz. turkey bacon cooked with olive oil, high-oleic (high-heat) sunflower oil, high-oleic (high-heat) safflower oil or avocado oil

Lunch:
- Low-carb, low-fat, high-protein pasta: Sprouted-grain spaghetti**, olive oil, low-sodium tomato sauce, ground chicken or turkey with Italian seasoning**

Dinner:
- Soft chicken tacos: 3-6 oz. shredded chicken, shredded lettuce, diced tomatoes, low-fat cheese and avocado on a sprouted-grain tortilla**

*Suggested whole-grain cereals: Fiber One, All Bran, Total, Cheerios. Fiber One and All Bran are my favorites because of the high fiber content.

** Go to www.eduardodias.com/resources for specialty items or anything you can't find easily in your grocery store.

29

WEEK 4 [Your own Menu]

MONDAY

Breakfast:
Protein:
Carb:
Fat:

Lunch:
Protein:
Carb:
Fat:

Dinner:
Protein:
Carb:
Fat:

TUESDAY

Breakfast:
Protein:
Carb:
Fat:

Lunch:
Protein:
Carb:
Fat:

Dinner:
Protein:
Carb:

WEDNESDAY

Breakfast:
Protein:
Carb:
Fat:

Lunch:
Protein:
Carb:
Fat:

Dinner:
Protein:
Carb:
Fat:

THURSDAY

Breakfast:
Protein:
Carb:
Fat:

Lunch:
Protein:
Carb:
Fat:

Dinner:
Protein:
Carb:
Fat:

FRIDAY

Breakfast:
Protein:
Carb:
Fat:

SATURDAY

Breakfast:
Protein:
Carb:
Fat:

Lunch:
Protein:
Carb:
Fat:

Dinner:
Protein:

SUNDAY

Breakfast:
Protein:
Carb:
Fat:

Lunch:
Protein:
Carb:
Fat:

EATING OUT

I used to say that eating out should be done only as a treat. However, I've learned that some people must eat out often, either because of work or simply because they don't like to prepare food.

I want you to succeed no matter what your lifestyle, so I am giving you one entire week of sample menus for dining out. Again, my goal is to give you an idea of how to adjust your meals. You'll still be having a substantial breakfast and lunch and a light dinner, and you'll still need to get the right quantities of protein and carbs and the right kinds of fats.

Most restaurants will have the items I'm suggesting. *Do not be shy about requesting the suggested adjustments.* As you get familiar with the plan, you will be able to make the best choices and right adjustments at virtually any type of restaurant.

EATING-OUT MENU

MONDAY

Breakfast:
- 1–2 eggs, any style, cooked with olive oil or no oil
- Turkey burger patty
- Small portion of hash browns or potatoes, preferably cooked with olive oil
- Add 1–2 Tbs. of olive oil to scrambled eggs or hash browns★

Lunch:
- Garden salad with low-fat dressing or vinegar and olive oil★
- Broiled, baked or grilled salmon
- Asparagus (if not available, mixed vegetables or any vegetable from the food table)
- If you didn't put olive oil or dressing on the salad, add 1–2 Tbs. of olive oil to the vegetables★

Dinner:
- Broiled, baked or grilled salmon
- Steamed vegetable mix with olive oil★

TUESDAY

Breakfast:
- Oatmeal
- Grilled chicken breast
- ½–1 avocado

Lunch:
- Grilled chicken-breast sandwich on ½ bun or 1 slice whole-grain bread with mustard or very light mayonnaise only
- Fruit salad (or any fruit from the food table)
- ½–1 avocado

Dinner:
- Cottage cheese, preferably low-fat
- 1 slice whole-grain toast with very light butter or jelly
- ¼–½ avocado

WEDNESDAY

Breakfast:
- Omelet: 2–3 eggs, spinach, turkey
- 1–2 slices whole-grain toast with very light butter or jelly
- Add 1–2 Tbs. of olive oil to omelet★

Lunch:
- 1–2 turkey burger patties or turkey slices (no gravy)
- Small portion of garbanzo beans or choice of beans
- Carrots
- Add 1–2 Tbs. of olive oil to carrots, beans or turkey★

Dinner:
- Salad: grilled chicken breast, lettuce, tomatoes, cucumbers, carrots, garbanzo beans with olive oil and vinegar★

THURSDAY

Breakfast:
- 1–2 eggs, any style, cooked with olive oil or no oil
- Whole-grain cereal with low fat milk★★
- Add 1–2 tablespoon of olive oil to eggs★

Lunch:
- Tuna sandwich on 1 slice whole-grain bread
- Steamed vegetables with olive oil★
- Garden salad with olive oil and vinegar★

Dinner:
- Turkey on 1 slice whole-grain bread with mustard or very light mayonnaise only
- ¼– ½ avocado

FRIDAY

Breakfast:
- Cottage cheese, preferably low-fat
- Fruit salad (or any fruit from the food table)
- ½–1 avocado

Lunch:
- Broiled, baked or grilled salmon
- ½ baked potato with olive oil and chives★
- Green beans (if not available, mixed vegetables or any vegetable from the food table)

Dinner:
- Greek salad: Romaine lettuce, tomatoes, cucumber, red onions, black olives and feta cheese with olive oil★

SATURDAY

Breakfast:
- 1–2 eggs, any style, cooked with olive oil or no oil
- Canadian bacon or ham
- 1–2 slices whole-grain toast with very little butter or jelly

Lunch:
- Turkey burger on ½ of a whole-grain bun with mustard or very light mayonnaise only
- Steamed vegetables with olive oil★
- Garden salad with olive oil and vinegar★

Dinner:
- Grilled freshwater trout (or any fish from the food table)

SUNDAY

Breakfast:
- Smoked salmon omelet: 2–3 eggs and smoked salmon
- Fruit salad (or any fruit from the food table)
- Add 1–2 Tbs. of olive oil to the omelet★

Lunch:
- Garden salad with low-fat dressing or vinegar and olive oil★
- Grilled chicken breast
- Spinach with olive oil (if not available, mixed vegetables or any vegetable from the food table)★

Dinner:
- Tuna sandwich on 1 slice whole-grain bread
- Steamed spinach (if not available, mixed vegetables or any vegetable from the food table) with olive oil★

★ Go to www.eduardodias.com/resources for web stores to buy olive oil packets in case the restaurant doesn't carry olive oil.

★★ Suggested whole-grain cereals: Fiber One, All Bran, Total, Cheerios. Fiber One and All Bran are my favorites because of the high fiber content.

Now go and make it happen!

You've read the eating plan that has helped each of my clients to achieve the body he or she has always dreamed of and to effortlessly keep it for life.

There is only one thing I cannot give you in this book: the desire and determination to achieve your goals. All I can do is remind you that you are strong and capable. I can guarantee you that, regardless of where you are in terms of weight and fitness level, you are a success in some parts of your life. Look at those successful areas of your life and let them guide and inspire you to achieve your health and weight-loss goals.

And brace for the journey. Be ready for changes, because they will happen.

If you once saw yourself as someone who struggles with weight, that is about to change. If you considered yourself someone who eats badly, that too will change. You may have been an unhealthy person, but you won't be for long.

Be prepared for that change. It can be frightening and exciting. Just know that the person you are changing into is happier and healthier. And I guarantee you that is worth the journey.

Also remember, a journey is rarely a straight upward line. There may be setbacks along the way, but if you keep at it, you will succeed.

Now go and make it happen. Be healthy, be fit, and have a great body!

Send me your success story.

Help inspire someone else. Send me your success story to post on my website and possibly to include in a future book. You could be an inspiration to millions of people all over the world!

Here's what to do:

- Send a **full-body** before and after photo to success@eduardodias.com with your name, address and phone number. Make sure the "after" photo is recent.

- Tell me your story; anything you want to share, including how much you weighed before and how much you weigh now, how long it took you to arrive at you current weight and any gold nuggets you would like to share. You may include your age.

To thank you for sharing, you will be entered in a monthly drawing to receive a free phone-coaching session with me.

Of course, I'm always open to receive your emails with questions, suggestions and input. I look forward to hearing from you.

Eduardo's Super Soup

3 lbs. of vegetables: spinach, asparagus, carrot, green beans, onion, cauliflower, broccoli, Brussels sprouts, celery, artichoke, bell pepper, mushroom, sprouts (any kind)

Low-sodium chicken broth (1 liter)

2 lbs. chicken (ground, diced or shredded)

Basil

Healthy Mayo

Eggs

Dijon mustard

Sea salt

High-oleic (high-heat) sunflower oil, high-oleic (high-heat) safflower oil or avocado oil

Lemon juice or white-wine vinegar

Berry Awesome Shake

Casein protein powder

1 % low-fat milk or almond milk

Berries (blueberries, raspberries, blackberries, strawberries or a mix of any of these)

Avocado Spread

Avocado (1 med.)

Onion (1)

Garlic (1)

Tomato (1)

Cilantro (1 bunch)

Lime juice (8 oz. or small size)

Chili powder

Sea salt

Avocado Spread, Short Version

Avocado (1 med.)

MSG-free seasoned salt

Salmon Paté

Fresh or canned salmon

Nonfat or low-fat cream cheese

Dill

Shopping List
Week 1

Dry Items (for all three weeks)

Sprouted-grain bread (1 loaf)
Sprouted-grain buns (1 package) **
Sprouted-grain English muffins (1 package) **
Sprouted-grain hot dog buns (1 package)**
Sprouted-grain pizza crust (1) **
Sprouted-grain tortillas (1 package)**
Sprouted-grain spaghetti **
Gnocchi
Dry oats (18 oz.)
Whole-grain cereal* (1 box)
Whole-grain pancake mix (6 oz.)
Black beans (1 lb.)
Garbanzo beans (1 lb.)
Pinto beans (1 lb.)
Wild rice (1 lb.)
Low-sodium tomato sauce (2 small cans)
Almonds (8 oz.)
Cashews (8 oz.)
Macadamia nuts (8 oz.)
Italian seasoning **
Mexican seasoning **
Low-fat salad dressing
Flax-seed oil
MSG-free seasoned salt
Olive oil
Stevia
High-oleic (high-heat) sunflower oil, high-oleic (high-heat) safflower oil or avocado oil

*Suggested whole-grain cereals: Fiber One, All Bran, Total, Cheerios. Fiber One and All Bran are my favorites because of the high fiber content.

** Go to www.eduardodias.com/resources for specialty items or anything that you can't find easily in your grocery store.

Dairy

Eggs (1 dozen)
1 % low-fat or almond milk (1/2 gallon carton or 2 quarts)
Low-fat cheese: American, Monterrey Jack, cheddar or Swiss (16 oz.; save remainder for weeks Two and Three)
Low-fat mozzarella (8 oz.)
Low-fat cottage cheese (8 oz.)

Produce

Asparagus (1 lb., separated; freeze remainder for week Three)
Bell pepper (1 med.)
Broccoli (1 small head or 1 bag, frozen; save remainder for weeks Two and Three)
Carrots (3 med.)
Cauliflower (1 small or 1 bag, frozen; save remainder for weeks Two and Three)
Celery (1 bunch)
Cucumber (1)
Green beans (5-8 oz. or 1 bag, frozen; save remainder for weeks Two and Three)
Mushrooms (5 oz.)
Onion (1)
Pearl onions (1 bag, frozen)
Potato, white (1 med.), or hash browns (16 oz.; save remainder for weeks Two and Three)
Romaine lettuce (1 head)
Spinach (1/2 bunch, fresh)
Tomatoes (2 med.)

Meat and Seafood

Chicken or turkey burger (1 lb., save remainder for weeks Two and Three)
Chicken breast (two breasts, 3-8 oz. each)
Freshwater trout or any fish from the food table (2-6 oz.)
Ground chicken or turkey (8 oz.-1 lb.)
Chicken or turkey breakfast sausage (3-5 oz.)
Lean carnitas (3-8 oz.)
Lean ham (2-6 oz.)
Lean pork chop (3-8 oz.)
Salmon (2 filets, 3-8 oz. each)
Tuna in olive oil (1 can)
Turkey bacon (8 oz. bag. Save leftover for week Two)
Turkey sausage (3-8 oz.)

Fruits

Avocados (3 med.)
Banana (1 med.)
Fruit salad (8 oz.)
Strawberries (8 oz.)

Shopping List
Week 2

Fruits

Apple (1 med.)

Avocado (3-5 med.)

Banana (1 med.)

Blueberries (5 oz.)

Strawberries (5 oz.)

Produce

Bell pepper (1 med.)

Carrots (3 med.)

Cucumber (1)

Mushrooms (5 oz.)

Potato, russet-for baking (1 small)

Potato, white (2 med.)

Hash browns (16 oz. or leftover from week One)

Spinach (1/2 bunch or 1 frozen bag and save leftover for week Three)

Romaine lettuce (2 heads)

Tomatoes (2 med.)

Zucchini (1 med.)

Meat and Seafood

Baby shrimp (2-6 oz.)

Canadian bacon (3-8 oz.)

Chicken or turkey burger (2 patties or remainder from week One)

Gourmet chicken sausage (3-8 oz.) **

Ground chicken or turkey (2-6 oz.)

Salmon (3-8 oz.)

Shrimp (3-8 oz.)

Lean hamburger, chicken or turkey burger (3-8 oz. or leftover from week One)

Lean pork chops (3- 8 oz.)

Lean steak (3-8 oz.)

Turkey bacon (2-4 oz.)

** Go to www.eduardodias.com/resources for specialty items or anything that you can't find easily in your grocery store.

Dairy

Eggs (12-18)

1 % low-fat milk or almond milk (1/2 gallon or 2 quarts)

Low-fat cheese: American, Monterrey Jack, cheddar, mozzarella or Swiss (8 oz. or remainder from week One)

Low-fat cottage cheese (8 oz.)

Low-fat plain yogurt (8 oz.)

Low-fat sour cream (8 oz.)

Shopping List
Week 3

Fruits

    Avocado (2-4 med.)

    Pear (1 med.)

    Fruit salad (8 oz.)

    Strawberries (8 oz.)

    Black olives (5 oz. fresh or 1 small can)

Produce

    Asparagus (1 lb. or remainder from week One)

    Carrots (2 med.)

    Cauliflower (1 small head or frozen leftover from week One)

    Cucumber (1)

    Mushrooms (5 oz.)

    Potato, white (2 med.)

    Hash browns (16 oz. or leftover from weeks One and Two)

    Spinach (1 bunch or frozen leftover from week Two)

    Red onion (1)

    Romaine lettuce (2 heads)

    Scallions (1 bunch)

    Tomatoes (3 med.)

Meat and Seafood

    Ahi tuna (3-8 oz.)

    Canadian bacon (2-4 oz.)

    Chicken breast (3-8oz.)

    Chicken or turkey burger (2 patties or remainder from weeks One and Two)

    Cod (3-8oz.)

    Ground chicken or turkey (6-12 oz.)

    Lean ham (3-6 oz.)

    Lean pork chops (3-8 oz.)

    Lean steak (3-8 oz.)

    Shredded chicken (3-6 oz.)

    Smoked salmon (3-8 oz.)

    Turkey (3-8 oz.)

    Turkey bacon (3-8 oz.)

Dairy

    Eggs (12-18)

    1 % low-fat milk or almond milk (1 quart)

    Low-fat cheese: American, Monterrey Jack, cheddar, mozzarella or Swiss (8 oz. or remainder from weeks One and Two)

    Low-fat cottage cheese (8 oz.)

    Feta cheese (8 oz.)

    Low-fat plain yogurt (16 oz.)

APPENDIX 2: *Resources/Where to buy*

Many of the "specialty items" I mention, such as sprouted-grain breads and gourmet chicken sausage, are available at health-food stores such as Whole Foods Market and Trader Joe's.

Also, links on my website take you to sites that sell all of the items on my plan. I constantly update this information. Many of these web stores give my clients a discount.

Visit www.eduardodias.com/resources.